American College of Surgeons
Protocol for Cancer Surgery Documentation: Pancreas Cancer

Name: ACS.CSSP.protocol.pancreas.2023.v1

What This Protocol Includes and Covers

- A synoptic operative report for pancreas cancer surgery
  - Section 1: EMR Autopopulated Information
  - Section 2: Cancer-Specific Information (required)
  - Section 3: Additional Procedure Details
- The synoptic operative report summary template
- Knowledge Platform with explanatory notes

American College of Surgeons Standards References

The following ACS standards references are heavily leveraged throughout the synoptic operative report and Knowledge Platform: *AJCC Cancer Staging Manual, Eighth Edition; Operative Standards for Cancer Surgery*, Volume 1; and *Standards for Oncology Registry Entry (STORE) 2023*.

Authors

William R. Burns, MD, FACS*; Matthew H. G. Katz, MD, FACS*; Elliot Newman, MD, FACS*; Peter Peng, MD, FACS*

Reviewers

Syed A. Ahmad, MD, FACS†; Melissa E. Hogg, MD, FACS†; Carmen C. Solorzano, MD, FACS†; Susan Tsai, MD, MHS, FACS†

Contributors

Peter Allen, MD, FACS; Waddah B. Al-Refaie, MD, FACS; M. Mura Assifi, MD, FACS; Adam C. Berger, MD, FACS; Mitchell Chorost, MD, FACS; Yun Shin Chun, MD, FACS; W. Charles Conway II, MD, FACS; Kristopher P. Croome, MD, FACS; Wendy L. Frankel, MD; Paul Hansen, MD, FACS; John P. Hoffman, MD, FACS; Kaitlyn Kelly, MD, FACS; Michael L. Kendrick, MD, FACS; Andrew M. Lowy, MD, FACS; Nipun Merchant, MD, FACS; William H. Nealon, MD, FACS; Timothy M. Pawlik, MD, MPH, PhD, FACS; Peter W.T. Pisters, MD, MHCM, FACS; Mitchell C. Posner, MD, FACS; Aaron R. Sasson, MD, FACS; Roderich E. Schwarz, MD, PhD, FACS; Brett C. Sheppard, MD, MS, FACS; Mark J. Truty, MD, MSc; Jennifer F. Tseng, MD, MPH, FACS; Caroline Verbeke, MD, PhD, FRCPath; Charles Vollmer, MD, FACS; Sharon M. Weber, MD, FACS; Emily Winslow, MD, FACS; Ronald Wolf, MD, FACS; Nicholas J. Zyromski, MD, FACS

**Denotes primary author. †Denotes synoptic operative report reviewer.*

Synoptic Operative Report

What This Synoptic Operative Report Includes and Covers
This synoptic operative report (SOR) covers pancreas cancer surgery documentation.
The SOR includes roughly 15–19 fields each for EMR autopopulated data, cancer-specific data *(required)*, and additional procedure data that assist with billing and regulatory and practice requirements. This synoptic operative report was designed for cases of pancreatic ductal adenocarcinoma and pancreatic neuroendocrine tumors and for pancreatoduodenectomy (Whipple procedure), distal subtotal pancreatectomy, total pancreatectomy, and local excision/ enucleation. It is not designed for cystic lesions nor central pancreatectomy; however, narrative text boxes may facilitate expanded use of this synoptic report at the user's discretion.

How This Synoptic Operative Report Is Organized
Required fields are indicated by an asterisk (*).

Section 1: EMR Autopopulated Information
Patient Name*
Patient ID*
Date of Surgery*
Name of Surgeon*
Name of Co-Surgeon
Name of Assistant(s)
Indication for Surgery*
Preoperative Diagnosis*
Postoperative Diagnosis*
Procedure(s) Performed*
Specimens Removed
Type of Anesthesia
Estimated Blood Loss
Drain/Implant
Additional Administrative Details

Section 2: Cancer-Specific Information
Preoperative Diagnosis*
Preoperative Histopathology*
Intent of Surgery*
Preoperative Tumor Location*
Radiographic Findings at Presentation*
Radiographic Classification of Primary Tumor Anatomy*
Tumor Marker(s)*
Preoperative Therapy*
Intraoperative Primary Tumor Findings, T Category*
Intraoperative Lymph Node Findings, N Category*
Intraoperative Metastatic Findings, M Category*
Extrapancreatic Disease*
Assessment and Management of Vascular Involvement by Tumor*
Aberrant Arterial Anatomy*
Completeness of Pancreatic Resection*
Intraoperative Margin Assessment*
Additional Intraoperative Pathology Specimens*
Procedure Performed*
Extent of Dissection and Lymphadenectomy*

Section 3: Additional Procedure Details

Staging Laparoscopy Performed
Operative Approach
Cholecystectomy
Extent of Gastric Resection
Orientation of Reconstruction
Pancreatic Reconstruction
Biliary Reconstruction
Intestinal Reconstruction
Splenectomy
Method of Pancreatic Transection
Management of Pancreatic 'Stump'
Drains
Stents
Additional Procedures
Additional Surgical Information
Intraoperative Complications

Instructions

This report is intended for documentation at the completion of each surgical procedure.

Instructions are provided for each data field.

Explanatory notes provide reference material for each data field.

Narrative boxes are available in all sections of the SOR to allow the addition of provider-specific information as needed.

Completing all applicable data fields in the SOR will generate a SOR summary that is compliant with multiple regulatory requirements.

- **Section 1 Instructions:** You are being asked to review all the data fields in Section 1 as the information is autopopulated from the EMR and should be checked for accuracy. Please make corrections as needed and be sure to complete required fields. Throughout the tool, required fields are marked with an asterisk (*) and represent best practice.
- **Section 2 Instructions:** You are asked to complete all data fields in this section (Cancer-Specific Information) because they are required as best practice.
- **Section 3 Instructions:** You are not required to complete these data fields, but the additional surgical data elements included in this section (Additional Procedure Details) will support diverse coding, regulatory, and practice needs.

Section 1: EMR Autopopulated Information (Note A)

Patient Name*
Patient ID*
Date of Surgery*
Name of Surgeon*
Name of Co-Surgeon
Name of Assistant(s)
Indication for Surgery*
Preoperative Diagnosis*
Postoperative Diagnosis*
Procedure(s) Performed*
Specimens Removed
Type of Anesthesia
Estimated Blood Loss
Drain/Implant
Additional Administrative Details

Section 2: Cancer-Specific Information (Note B)

Preoperative Assessment

*** Preoperative Diagnosis** (Note C)
Select single best answer.
__ Pancreatic ductal adenocarcinoma [*Narrative Box*]
__ Pancreatic neuroendocrine tumor [*Narrative Box*]
__ Other [*Narrative Box*]

*** Preoperative Histopathology** (Note D)
Has preoperative diagnosis been confirmed by histopathology? Select single best answer.
__ Yes
__ No

*** Intent of Surgery** (Note E)
Was the operation performed for curative intent? Select single best answer.
__ Yes
__ No

If no:
Select single best answer.
__ Diagnostic intent [*Narrative Box*]
__ Staging intent [*Narrative Box*]
__ Palliative intent [*Narrative Box*]

*** Preoperative Tumor Location** (Note F)
For a solitary lesion, select single best answer. For multiple lesions, select all that apply.
__ Head of pancreas (including uncinate)
__ Neck of pancreas (or other specified parts of pancreas)
__ Body of pancreas
__ Tail of pancreas
__ Single overlapping lesion across any pancreas region above

*** Radiographic Findings at Presentation** (Note G)
Select single best answer.
__ Cancer localized to the pancreas without radiographic evidence for major vascular involvement or regional lymphadenopathy
__ Cancer localized to the pancreas with radiographic evidence for major vascular involvement and/or regional lymphadenopathy
__ Radiographic evidence for distant metastasis

*** Radiographic Classification of Primary Tumor Anatomy** (Note H)
Select single best answer.
__ Resectable
__ Borderline resectable
__ Locally advanced

*** Tumor Marker(s)** (Note I)
Which preoperative tumor markers were obtained? Select all that apply.
__ None
__ Serum CA19-9 preoperative value: _____ U/mL
__ Chromogranin A: ____ ng/mL
__ CEA: ____ ng/mL
__ Other—Specify [*Narrative Box*]

*** Preoperative Therapy** (Note J)
Select all that apply.
__ None
__ Systemic therapy (including chemotherapy, targeted therapy, immunotherapy, endocrine [hormonal] therapy, etc.)
__ Radiation therapy (including chemoradiation)
__ Other/Comments [*Narrative Box*]

Intraoperative Findings

[If "Pancreatic ductal adenocarcinoma" was selected under ***Preoperative Diagnosis****, display the following three fields:]*

*** Intraoperative Primary Tumor Findings, T Category** (Note K)
Select single best answer.
__ Primary tumor does not appear to involve celiac axis, superior mesenteric artery, and/or common hepatic artery (T1/T2/T3)

__ Primary tumor appears to involve celiac axis, superior mesenteric artery, and/or common hepatic artery (T4)
[If "Primary tumor appears to involve celiac axis, superior mesenteric artery, and/or common hepatic artery (T4)" is selected, display the following:]
Select all that apply.
__ Celiac axis
__ Superior mesenteric artery
__ Common hepatic artery
__ Primary tumor cannot be assessed (TX)

*** Intraoperative Lymph Node Findings, N Category** (Note L)
Select single best answer.
__ No suspected adenopathy (N0)
__ Suspected regional adenopathy (N1-N2)
[If "Suspected regional adenopathy (N1-N2)" is selected, display the following:]
Select single best answer.
__ Completely resected
__ Not completely resected [*Narrative Box*]
__ Regional lymph nodes cannot be assessed (NX)

*** Intraoperative Metastatic Findings, M Category** (Note M)
Select single best answer.
__ No suspected distant metastasis (M0)
__ Suspected distant metastasis (M1)
[If "Suspected distant metastasis (M1)" is selected, display the following:]
Select all that apply.
__ Findings suspicious for extraregional adenopathy
__ Findings suspicious for peritoneal carcinomatosis
__ Findings suspicious for liver metastasis
__ Findings suspicious for metastasis to other distant organ [*Narrative Box*]

[If "Pancreatic neuroendocrine tumor" was selected under ***Preoperative Diagnosis****, display the following three fields:]*
*** Intraoperative Primary Tumor Findings, T Category** (Note K)
Select single best answer.
__ Primary tumor appears limited to the pancreas measuring up to 4 cm with/without extension into peripancreatic adipose tissue (T1/T2)
__ Primary tumor appears limited to the pancreas measuring greater than 4 cm with/without extension into peripancreatic adipose tissue; or primary tumor invading the duodenum or common bile duct (T3)
[If "Primary tumor appears limited to the pancreas measuring greater than 4 cm with/without extension into peripancreatic adipose tissue; or primary tumor invading the duodenum or common bile duct (T3)" is selected, display the following:]
Select all that apply.
__ Primary tumor appears limited to the pancreas measuring greater than 4 cm with/without extension into peripancreatic adipose tissue
__ Primary tumor appears to be invading the duodenum or common bile duct
__ Primary tumor appears to be invading other adjacent organs or major arteries (T4)
[If "Primary tumor appears to be invading other adjacent organs or major arteries (T4)" is selected, display the following:]
Select all that apply.
__ Stomach
__ Spleen
__ Colon
__ Adrenal gland
__ Other adjacent organ [*Narrative Box*]
__ Celiac axis
__ Superior mesenteric artery
__ Primary tumor cannot be assessed (TX)

*** Intraoperative Lymph Node Findings, N Category** (Note L)
Select single best answer.
__ No suspected adenopathy (N0)
__ Suspected regional adenopathy (N1)
[If "Suspected regional adenopathy (N1)" is selected, display the following:]
Select single best answer.
__ Completely resected
__ Not completely resected [*Narrative Box*]
__ Regional lymph nodes cannot be assessed (NX)

* Intraoperative Metastatic Findings, M Category (Note M)
Select single best answer.
__ No suspected distant metastasis (M0)
__ Suspected metastasis confined to liver (M1a)
__ Suspected metastasis confined to at least one extrahepatic site (M1b)
[If "Suspected metastasis confined to at least one extrahepatic site (M1b)" is selected, display the following:]
Select all that apply.
__ Findings suspicious for extraregional adenopathy
__ Findings suspicious for peritoneal carcinomatosis
__ Findings suspicious for ovarian metastasis
__ Findings suspicious for metastasis to other distant organ [*Narrative Box*]
__ Suspected hepatic and extrahepatic metastases (M1c)
[If "Suspected hepatic and extrahepatic metastases (M1c)" is selected, display the following:]
Select all that apply.
__ Findings suspicious for extraregional adenopathy
__ Findings suspicious for peritoneal carcinomatosis
__ Findings suspicious for ovarian metastasis
__ Findings suspicious for metastasis to other distant organ [*Narrative Box*]

*** Extrapancreatic Disease** (Note N)
Select single best answer.
__ No
__ Yes
[If "Yes" is selected, display the following:]
Select all that apply.
__ Peritoneum
__ Liver
__ Other [*Narrative Box*]

*** Assessment and Management of Vascular Involvement by Tumor** (Note O)
Select all vessels that were assessed.
__ Portal vein
[If "Portal vein" is selected, display the following:]
Select single best answer.
__ No contact
__ Separable
__ Inseparable
[If "Inseparable" is selected, display the following:]
Management of Vascular Involvement
Select single best answer.
__ Tangential without patch [*Narrative Box*]
__ Tangential with patch [*Narrative Box*]
__ Segmental without graft [*Narrative Box*]
__ Segmental with graft [*Narrative Box*]
__ Superior mesenteric vein
[If "Superior mesenteric vein" is selected, display the following:]
Select single best answer.
__ No contact
__ Separable
__ Inseparable
[If "Inseparable" is selected, display the following:]
Management of Vascular Involvement
Select single best answer.
__ Tangential without patch [*Narrative Box*]
__ Tangential with patch [*Narrative Box*]
__ Segmental without graft [*Narrative Box*]
__ Segmental with graft [*Narrative Box*]
__ Superior mesenteric artery
[If "Superior mesenteric artery" is selected, display the following:]
Select single best answer.
__ No contact
__ Separable
__ Inseparable
[If "Inseparable" is selected, display the following:]
Management of Vascular Involvement
Select single best answer.
__ Tangential without patch [*Narrative Box*]
__ Tangential with patch [*Narrative Box*]
__ Segmental without graft [*Narrative Box*]
__ Segmental with graft [*Narrative Box*]
__ Hepatic artery
[If "Hepatic artery" is selected, display the following:]
Select single best answer.
__ No contact
__ Separable
__ Inseparable
[If "Inseparable" is selected, display the following:]
Management of Vascular Involvement
Select single best answer.
__ Tangential without patch [*Narrative Box*]
__ Tangential with patch [*Narrative Box*]
__ Segmental without graft [*Narrative Box*]
__ Segmental with graft [*Narrative Box*]

__ Celiac trunk:
[If "Celiac trunk" is selected, display the following:]
Select single best answer.
__ No contact
__ Separable
__ Inseparable
[If "Inseparable" is selected, display the following:]
Management of Vascular Involvement
Select single best answer.
__ Tangential without patch [*Narrative Box*]
__ Tangential with patch [*Narrative Box*]
__ Segmental without graft [*Narrative Box*]
__ Segmental with graft [*Narrative Box*]
__ Other vessels—Describe assessment and management of vascular involvement by tumor [**Narrative Box*]

*** Aberrant Arterial Anatomy** (Note P)
Select single best answer.
__ No
__ Yes—Specify [**Narrative Box*]

*** Completeness of Pancreatic Resection** (Note Q)
Select single best answer.
__ R0/R1
__ R2 [*Narrative Box*]

*** Intraoperative Margin Assessment** (Note R)
Select all that apply.
__ None
__ Pancreatic parenchymal margin
[If "Pancreatic parenchymal margin" is selected, display the following:]
Select single best answer.
__ Positive
__ Negative
__ Bile duct margin
[If "Bile duct margin" is selected, display the following:]
Select single best answer.
__ Positive
__ Negative
__ Uncinate (retroperitoneal/superior mesenteric artery) margin
[If "Uncinate margin" is selected, display the following:]
Select single best answer.
__ Positive
__ Negative
__ Other [**Narrative Box*]

*** Additional Intraoperative Pathology Specimens** (Note S)
Select single best answer.
__ None
__ Yes—Describe [**Narrative Box*]

*** Procedure Performed** (Note T)
Select single best answer.
__ Pancreatoduodenectomy (Whipple procedure)
__ Distal subtotal pancreatectomy
__ Total pancreatectomy
__ Local excision/enucleation

*** Extent of Dissection and Lymphadenectomy** (Note U)
Select single best answer for each category.

[If "Pancreatoduodenectomy" or "Total pancreatectomy" was selected above, display the following:]
Plane of Uncinate (Retroperitoneal/Superior Mesenteric Artery) Dissection
__ Periadventitial dissection of superior mesenteric artery
__ Alternate plane of retroperitoneal dissection

[If "Distal subtotal pancreatectomy" or "Total pancreatectomy" was selected above, display the following:]
Plane of Posterior Dissection
__ Superficial to retroperitoneal fascia
__ Alternate plane of posterior dissection

[If "Pancreatoduodenectomy" or "Distal subtotal pancreatectomy" was selected above, display the following:]
Site of Pancreatic Transection
__ Pancreatic neck
__ Alternate site of pancreatic transection [*Narrative Box*]

[If "Local excision/enucleation" was selected above, display the following:]
Preservation of Main Pancreatic Duct
__ Yes
__ No—Explain [*Narrative Box*]

Extent of Lymphadenectomy
__ Standard for pancreatoduodenectomy (peripancreatic nodes, porta hepatis nodes, and right lateral aspect of superior mesenteric artery nodes)
__ Standard for distal subtotal pancreatectomy (peripancreatic nodes, splenic hilum)
__ Standard for total pancreatectomy (peripancreatic nodes, porta hepatis nodes, and right lateral aspect of superior mesenteric artery nodes, splenic hilum)
__ Alternate or local excision/enucleation—Select all nodal basins that apply:
    __ Peripancreatic (head and uncinate process)
    __ Porta hepatis
    __ Superior mesenteric artery (right lateral aspect only)
    __ Para-aortic
    __ Peripancreatic (body and tail)
    __ Splenic hilum

Other Noteworthy Findings
__ None
__ Yes—Describe [**Narrative Box*]

Section 3: Additional Procedure Details (Note V)

Staging Laparoscopy Performed (Note W)
Select single best answer.
__ Yes
__ No

Operative Approach (Note X)
Select single best answer.
__ Open
__ Laparoscopic
__ Robotic
__ Other [**Narrative Box*]

[If "Pancreatoduodenectomy" was selected under ***Procedure Performed****, display the following six fields:]*

Cholecystectomy (Note Y)
Select single best answer.
__ Yes
__ No

Extent of Gastric Resection (Note Z)
Select single best answer.
__ Classic (Distal gastrectomy)
__ Pylorus preserving

Orientation of Reconstruction (Note AA)
Select single best answer.
__ Loop (Billroth II type) [*Narrative Box*]
__ Roux-en-Y [*Narrative Box*]
__ Other [*Narrative Box*]

Pancreatic Reconstruction (Note BB)
Select single best answer.
__ Pancreaticojejunostomy
[If "Pancreaticojejunostomy" is selected, display the following:]
Select single best answer.
__ One-layer duct-to-mucosa [*Narrative Box*]
__ Two-layer duct-to-mucosa [*Narrative Box*]
__ Pancreatic invagination [*Narrative Box*]
__ Other [*Narrative Box*]
__ Pancreaticogastrostomy
[If "Pancreaticogastrostomy" is selected, display the following:]
Select single best answer.
__ One-layer duct-to-mucosa [*Narrative Box*]
__ Two-layer duct-to-mucosa [*Narrative Box*]
__ Pancreatic invagination [*Narrative Box*]
__ Other [*Narrative Box*]
__ Other [*Narrative Box*]
__ No reconstruction

Biliary Reconstruction (Note CC)
Select single best answer.
__ One-layer duct-to-mucosa [*Narrative Box*]
__ Other [*Narrative Box*]

Intestinal Reconstruction (Note DD)
Select single best answer.
__ Gastrojejunostomy
[If "Gastrojejunostomy" is selected, display the following:]
Select single best answer.
__ Stapled [*Narrative Box*]
__ Hand-sewn [*Narrative Box*]
__ Other [*Narrative Box*]
__ Duodenojejunostomy
[If "Duodenojejunostomy" is selected, display the following:]
Select single best answer.
__ Stapled [*Narrative Box*]
__ Hand-sewn [*Narrative Box*]
__ Other [*Narrative Box*]
__ Other [*Narrative Box*]

*[If "Distal subtotal pancreatectomy" was selected under **Procedure Performed**, display the following three fields:]*

Splenectomy (Note EE)
Select single best answer.
__ Yes
__ No

Method of Pancreatic Transection (Note FF)
Select single best answer.
__ Non-stapled [*Narrative Box*]
__ Stapled [*Narrative Box*]
__ Other [*Narrative Box*]

Management of Pancreatic 'Stump' (Note GG)
Select single best answer.
__ Suture [*Narrative Box*]
__ Stapled [*Narrative Box*]
__ None
__ Other [Narrative Box]

*[If "Total pancreatectomy" was selected under **Procedure Performed**, display the following five fields:]*

Cholecystectomy (Note Y)
Select single best answer.
__ Yes
__ No

Splenectomy (Note EE)
Select single best answer.
__ Yes
__ No

Extent of Gastric Resection (Note Z)
Select single best answer.
__ Classic (Distal gastrectomy)
__ Pylorus preserving

Biliary Reconstruction (Note CC)
Select single best answer.
__ One-layer duct-to-mucosa [*Narrative Box*]
__ Other [*Narrative Box*]

Intestinal Reconstruction (Note DD)
Select single best answer.
__ Gastrojejunostomy
[If "Gastrojejunostomy" is selected, display the following:]
Select single best answer.
__ Stapled [*Narrative Box*]
__ Hand-sewn [*Narrative Box*]
__ Other [*Narrative Box*]
__ Duodenojejunostomy
[If "Duodenojejunostomy" is selected, display the following:]
Select single best answer.
__ Stapled [*Narrative Box*]
__ Hand-sewn [*Narrative Box*]
__ Other [*Narrative Box*]
__ Other [*Narrative Box*]

Drains (Note HH)
Select single best answer.
__ Yes [*Narrative Box*]
__ No

Stents (Note II)
Select single best answer.
__ Yes [*Narrative Box*]
__ No

Additional Procedures (Note JJ)
Select single best answer.
__ Yes [**Narrative Box*]
__ No

Additional Surgical Information (Note KK)
Select single best answer.
__ Yes [**Narrative Box*]
__ No

Intraoperative Complications (Note LL)
Select single best answer.
__ Yes [**Narrative Box*]
__ No

Synoptic Operative Report Summary Template (Mockup)

Pancreas Cancer

Patient Name: *[Autopopulate from EMR]*
Patient ID: *[Autopopulate from EMR]*
Date of Surgery: *[Autopopulate from EMR]*
Name of Surgeon: *[Autopopulate from EMR]*
Name of Co-Surgeon: *[Autopopulate from EMR]*
Name of Assistant(s): *[Autopopulate from EMR – Nurses notes]*
Indication for Surgery: *[Autopopulate from EMR; **or** override with EMR pick list]*
Preoperative Diagnosis: *[Autopopulate from EMR; **or** override with SOR selections]*
Postoperative Diagnosis: *[Autopopulate from EMR; **or** override with SOR selections]*
Procedure(s) Performed: *[Autopopulate from EMR; **or** override with SOR selections]*
Specimens Removed: *[Autopopulate from EMR – Nurses notes with override capability]*
Type of Anesthesia: *[Autopopulate from EMR – Anesthesia with override capability]*
Estimated Blood Loss: *[Autopopulate from EMR – Anesthesia with override capability]*
Drain/Implant *[Autopopulate from EMR – Nurses notes with override capability]*
Additional Administrative Details: *[Autopopulate from EMR; **or** Narrative text]*

Cancer-Specific Information:
Preoperative Assessment

[Fill from SOR: Preoperative Diagnosis]
[Fill from SOR: Preoperative Histopathology]
[Fill from SOR: Intent of Surgery]
[Fill from SOR: Preoperative Tumor Location]
[Fill from SOR: Radiographic Findings at Presentation]
[Fill from SOR: Radiographic Classification of Primary Tumor Anatomy]
[Fill from SOR: Tumor Marker(s)]
[Fill from SOR: Preoperative Therapy]

Intraoperative Findings

[Fill from SOR: Intraoperative Primary Tumor Findings, T Category]
[Fill from SOR: Intraoperative Lymph Node Findings, N Category]
[Fill from SOR: Intraoperative Metastatic Findings, M Category]
[Fill from SOR: Extrapancreatic Disease]
[Fill from SOR: Assessment and Management of Vascular Involvement by Tumor]
[Fill from SOR: Aberrant Arterial Anatomy]
[Fill from SOR: Completeness of Pancreatic Resection]
[Fill from SOR: Intraoperative Margin Assessment]
[Fill from SOR: Additional Intraoperative Pathology Specimens]
[Fill from SOR: Procedure Performed]
[Fill from SOR: Extent of Dissection and Lymphadenectomy]

Additional Procedure Details (Page 2)

[Fill from SOR: Staging Laparoscopy Performed]
[Fill from SOR: Operative Approach]
[Fill from SOR as applicable: Cholecystectomy, Extent of Gastric Resection, Orientation of Reconstruction, Pancreatic Reconstruction, Biliary Reconstruction, Intestinal Reconstruction, Splenectomy, Method of Pancreatic Transection, and Management of Pancreatic 'Stump']
[Fill from SOR: Drains]
[Fill from SOR: Stents]
[Fill from SOR: Additional Procedures, Additional Surgical Information, and Intraoperative Complications]

Knowledge Platform

Introductory Comments:
This protocol is intended to standardize documentation and communication of critical components of surgery for pancreatic tumors. The following explanatory notes reference critical elements for cancer surgery as described in the *Operative Standards for Cancer Surgery*, Volume 1.

Instructions

Each Explanatory Note is linked from a corresponding data element in the synoptic report above and contains additional materials and references that can be used to facilitate accurate completion of the report.

Section 1: EMR Autopopulated Information

Note A: EMR Autopopulated Information

Explanatory Comments: The following fields are intended to be prepopulated with site-specific identifiers and information from the EMR.

Patient Name
Patient ID
Date of Surgery
Name of Surgeon
Name of Co-Surgeon
Name of Assistant(s)
Indication for Surgery
Preoperative Diagnosis
Postoperative Diagnosis
Procedure(s) Performed
Specimens Removed
Type of Anesthesia
Estimated Blood Loss
Drain/Implant
Additional Administrative Details

The following table (Table 1) contains the initial FHIR mappings for data fields in section 1, which can be used to create auto-population functionality. Note that FHIR mappings may vary by site and electronic health record (EHR) and will be revised over time.

Table 1. Data Field FHIR Mappings – Pancreas Cancer *(Untested)*

SOR Fields	Resource Main Category	Mapping	Version 4.0	Filter Codes Type	Filter Codes	Resource Link	Additional Links
Patient Name	Individual	patient.name	R4			https://fhir.cerner.com/millennium/r4/individuals/patient/	
MRN	Individual	patient.id	R4			https://fhir.cerner.com/millennium/r4/individuals/patient/	
Date of Surgery	Procedure	Procedure.performed[x]	R4	ICD 10 Procedure	N/A	https://hl7.org/fhir/R4/procedure-definitions.html#Procedure.encounter	See Choice of Data Types for further information about how [x] is used
Name of Surgeon	Scheduling	Appointment.participant.required	R4	SNOMED	1421009-766788081000087100	http://hl7.org/fhir/R4/appointment-definitions.html#Appointment.participant.actor	
Name of Co-Surgeon	Scheduling	Appointment.participant.required	R4	SNOMED	1421009-766788081000087100	http://hl7.org/fhir/R4/appointment-definitions.html#Appointment.participant.actor	
Name of Assistant(s)	Scheduling	Appointment.participant.required	R4	SNOMED	1421009-766788081000087100	http://hl7.org/fhir/R4/appointment-definitions.html#Appointment.participant.actor	
Indication for Surgery	Procedure	Procedure.reasoncode	R4	ICD10	0F1, 0F2, 0F5, 0F7, 0F8, 0F9, 0FB, 0FC, 0FD, 0FF, 0FH, 0FJ, 0FL, 0FM, 0FN, 0FP, 0FQ, 0FR, 0FS, 0FT, 0FU, 0FV, 0FW, 0FY	https://hl7.org/fhir/R4/procedure-definitions.html#Procedure.encounter	
Preoperative Diagnosis (ICD10)	Condition	Condition.Code	R4	ICD10	C25, D13, Q45, K86, S36	https://hl7.org/fhir/r4/condition-definitions.html#Condition.code	https://hl7.org/fhir/r4/valueset-condition-code.html
Postoperative Diagnosis (ICD10)	Condition	Condition.Code	R4	ICD10	C25, D13, Q45, K86, S36	https://hl7.org/fhir/r4/condition-definitions.html#Condition.code	
Procedure Performed	Procedure	Procedure.Code	R4	ICD10	0F1, 0F2, 0F5, 0F7, 0F8, 0F9, 0FB, 0FC, 0FD, 0FF, 0FH, 0FJ, 0FL, 0FM, 0FN, 0FP, 0FQ, 0FR, 0FS, 0FT, 0FU, 0FV, 0FW, 0FY	https://hl7.org/fhir/R4/valueset-procedure-code.html	

Specimens Removed	Observation Procedure	Observation. specimen Diagnostic Report.specimen	R4	ICD 10 Procedure	0F1, 0F2, 0F5, 0F7, 0F8, 0F9, 0FB, 0FC, 0FD, 0FF, 0FH, 0FJ, 0FL, 0FM, 0FN, 0FP, 0FQ, 0FR, 0FS, 0FT, 0FU, 0FV, 0FW, 0FY	https://hl7.org/fhir/R4/procedure-definitions.html#Procedure.reasonReference	https://hl7.org/fhir/R4/observation-definitions.html#Observation.value_x_
Type of Anesthesia	Diagnostic	Observation. code	R4	LOINC	10213-7	https://hl7.org/fhir/R4/valueset-observation-codes.html	
Estimated Blood Loss	Diagnostic	Observation. value	R4	LOINC	59770-8	https://hl7.org/fhir/R4/observation-definitions.html#Observation.value_x_	
Drain/Implant	Procedure	Procedure. focalDevice	R4	ICD 10 Procedure	0F9, 0FH	https://hl7.org/fhir/R4/observation-definitions.html#Observation.value_x_	
Additional Administrative Details	N/A	N/A					
Surgery Location (hidden field)	Procedure	Encounter. location				https://hl7.org/fhir/r4/encounter-definitions.html#Encounter.location	

Section 2: Cancer-Specific Information

Note B: Cancer-Specific Information

Explanatory Comments: This section of the synoptic operative report contains critical oncology data elements supported by evidence and best practice, as well as data fields defined by the STORE manual and submitted to hospital registries for NCDB and state registry reporting.

There are data fields in this section related to findings and/or treatments in both the preoperative and intraoperative phases of care. To complete the preoperative data fields assumes that the patient has undergone diagnostic imaging of the chest, abdomen, and pelvis to characterize the size, location, and vascular contact of the primary tumor, as well as the presence of regional or distant metastasis. For additional details, please refer to the *Operative Standards for Cancer Surgery,* Volume 2, pages 182–186.

Note C: Preoperative Diagnosis

Explanatory Comments: This protocol pertains to pancreatic ductal adenocarcinoma (pancreatic cancer) or pancreatic neuroendocrine (islet cell) tumors, and not, for example, benign or non-invasive pancreatic lesions. The preoperative cancer type should be selected based on microscopic confirmation of the diagnosis or suspected diagnosis based on preoperative testing. Histologic subtypes of pancreatic cancer (e.g., adenosquamous) should be documented within the narrative box for pancreatic adenocarcinoma. Likewise, whether tumors are functional (insulinoma, etc.) or non-functional should be documented within the narrative box for pancreatic neuroendocrine tumor.

Note D: Preoperative Histopathology

Explanatory Comments: This synoptic report is intended for use in all cases where there is reasonable clinical suspicion that the patient has a pancreatic tumor, even if the histopathology does not confirm the diagnosis preoperatively. To adjudicate any ambiguity in classification of tumors, please refer to the WHO histology classification of tumors codes listed in the *AJCC Cancer Staging Manual, Eighth Edition*, Chapter 28 (Exocrine Pancreas) and Chapter 34 (Neuroendocrine Tumors of the Pancreas).

Note E: Intent of Surgery

Explanatory Comments: Intent should be assigned postoperatively by the operating surgeon on the basis of preoperative evaluation and intraoperative management and should be documented as part of the operative report. Curative operations generally include complete resection of the primary tumor and regional lymphadenectomy for therapeutic or staging purposes. If the operation was not performed for curative intent, response options are provided for diagnostic, staging, or palliative intent along with narrative boxes to record any additional information.

Note F: Preoperative Tumor Location

Explanatory Comments: Tumor location and/or identification of synchronous tumors is important for surgical planning and is typically determined by preoperative imaging, sometimes aided by endoscopic ultrasonography. Understanding that intraoperative findings may alter the tumor location and extent of disease, tumor location should be indicated *based on preoperative imaging* by selecting a single best answer for a solitary lesion or selecting all answers that apply for multiple lesions.

NCDB coding instructions for *Primary Site* [400] are detailed in the STORE 2023 Manual. The primary site is recorded as a "C" preceding the three-digit code number (see Table 2). Overlapping lesion of pancreas (C258) can be used for single tumors that overlap the boundaries of two or more sub-sites and the point of origin is not known. Pancreas, NOS (C259) can be used for multiple tumors that originate in different subsites of one organ.

Table 2. Relevant NCDB Codes for Primary Site for Pancreatic Tumors

NCDB Code	Definition
C250	Head of pancreas
C251	Body of pancreas
C252	Tail of pancreas
C257	Other specified part of pancreas
C258	Overlapping lesion of pancreas

*This table is limited to the scope of this synoptic operative report and does not reflect an exhaustive list of primary site codes for the pancreas.

Note G: Radiographic Findings at Presentation

Explanatory Comments: Using diagnostic imaging to assess the extent of disease is important in multidisciplinary treatment planning. Specifically, radiographic evidence of vascular involvement, extent of regional adenopathy, or suspicion of distant metastasis will impact the treatment plan. Please select the best option based on initial staging workup (*at the time of presentation/diagnosis)* using the following guidance:

- Cancer localized to the pancreas is defined as tumor confined to the pancreas with or without surrounding retroperitoneal soft tissue or regional lymphadenopathy.
- Major vascular involvement is defined as tumor contact along the critical peripancreatic blood vessels (portal vein, superior mesenteric vein, celiac artery, hepatic artery, superior mesenteric artery, etc.)
- Regional lymphadenopathy is defined as grossly enlarged lymph nodes in one or more regional nodal basins or suspicious lymph nodes throughout multiple regional nodal basins.
    - Regional lymph nodes for tumors in the head or uncinate process of the pancreas include: peripancreatic, porta hepatis, superior mesenteric artery.
    - Regional lymph nodes for tumors in the body or tail of the pancreas include: peripancreatic, splenic hilum.
- Distant metastasis is defined as tumor spread to other organs or to lymph nodes outside the nodal basins mentioned above.

Note H: Radiographic Classification of Primary Tumor Anatomy

Explanatory Comments: The radiographic classification of the primary tumor anatomy is commonly used to describe resectability of the primary tumor and may be important in multidisciplinary treatment planning. This classification includes information not specifically captured in AJCC clinical staging but has particular relevance to surgeons. For example, this classification is often used to define populations of patients with pancreatic tumors receiving different treatments. Radiographic classification of the primary tumor should be recorded in this field based on established criteria summarized in the National Comprehensive Cancer Network (NCCN) Guidelines.

Pancreatic tumors that involve major vascular structures have a low likelihood of resectability and a high chance of incomplete removal if resected. Therefore, the Americas Hepato-Pancreato-Biliary Association/Society of Surgical Oncology/Society for Surgery of the Alimentary Tract, the International Study Group of Pancreatic Surgery (ISGPS), and the NCCN have defined criteria for "resectable", "borderline resectable", and "locally advanced" pancreatic tumors.

Resectable tumors have no contact with the celiac artery, hepatic artery, or superior mesenteric artery. Furthermore, there is no contour irregularity of the superior mesenteric vein or portal vein.

Borderline resectable tumors have some contact with the celiac artery, hepatic artery, superior mesenteric artery, superior mesenteric vein, and/or portal vein. The superior mesenteric artery may have tumor abutment up to but not more than 180 degrees of the circumference of the vessel and may have short segment involvement of the hepatic artery that does not extend onto the celiac axis. Venous involvement of the superior mesenteric vein/portal vein is defined as tumor abutment with or without impingement and narrowing of the lumen or short-segment venous occlusion resulting from either tumor thrombus or encasement but with suitable vessel proximal and distal to the area of vessel involvement.

Locally advanced tumors have extensive contact with the celiac artery, hepatic artery, superior mesenteric artery, superior mesenteric vein, and/or portal vein. Arterial involvement can include tumor encasement of the superior mesenteric artery or celiac axis by greater than 180 degrees of the circumference of the vessel or has encasement of the hepatic artery that does not allow for safe and complete resection and reconstruction. The extent of venous involvement is defined as encasement or occlusion of the superior mesenteric vein/portal vein that precludes reconstruction.

Note I: Tumor Marker(s)

Explanatory Comments: Tumor markers can be useful prognostic tools for pancreas cancer, and any preoperative tumor markers that were obtained should be documented here. Response options are listed for serum CA19-9, chromogranin A, and CEA, and blanks are provided to record the results for the markers that are selected. Other tumor markers not listed, such as pancreatic polypeptide, can be recorded using the "Other" field and associated narrative box.

Note J: Preoperative Therapy

Explanatory Comments: It is important to assess the tumor's response to preoperative chemotherapy and/or radiation therapy. For patients with borderline resectable or locally advanced cancers, preoperative therapy prior to surgical resection is the preferred treatment approach. Chemotherapy and/or chemoradiation may also be used to treat patients with resectable pancreatic ductal adenocarcinoma. Response options are provided for systemic therapy (which includes chemotherapy, targeted therapy, immunotherapy, and endocrine [hormonal] therapy) as well as radiation therapy (which includes chemoradiation). Other therapies can be recorded using the "Other" field and associated narrative box. For additional details, please refer to the *Operative Standards for Cancer Surgery*, Volume 1, pages 182–184.

Note K: Intraoperative Primary Tumor Findings, T Category

Explanatory Comments: In the context of intraoperative findings in this protocol for cancer surgery documentation, TNM categories from the American Joint Committee on Cancer (AJCC) are not designated with clinical (lower case "c" prefix) nor pathological (lower case "p" prefix) classifications. Determination of pathological classification involves a synthesis of information from multiple sources including clinical staging, operative findings, and pathological evaluation of resected surgical specimen(s). Complete information on TNM categories, clinical/pathological classifications, and the overall process of cancer staging can be found in the *AJCC Cancer Staging Manual, Eighth Edition.*

This field seeks to document intraoperative findings pertaining to whether the primary tumor is confined to the pancreas and, if not, the extent of the organ/venous involvement. These findings help inform pathological classification (see Table 3).

Table 3. Definition of Primary Tumor (T)

T Category	T Criteria (Exocrine Pancreas)	T Criteria (Neuroendocrine Tumors of the Pancreas)
TX	Primary tumor cannot be assessed	Tumor cannot be assessed
T1	Tumor ≤2 cm in greatest dimension	Tumor limited to the pancreas,* <2 cm
T2	Tumor >2 cm and ≤4 cm in greatest dimension	Tumor limited to the pancreas,* 2–4 cm
T3	Tumor >4 cm in greatest dimension	Tumor limited to the pancreas,* >4 cm; or tumor invading the duodenum or common bile duct
T4	Tumor involves celiac axis, superior mesenteric artery, and/or common hepatic artery, regardless of size	Tumor invading adjacent organs (stomach, spleen, colon, adrenal gland) or the wall of large vessels (celiac axis or the superior mesenteric artery)

**Limited to the pancreas means there is no invasion of adjacent organs (stomach, spleen, colon, adrenal gland) or the wall of large vessels (celiac axis or the superior mesenteric artery). Extension of tumor into peripancreatic adipose tissue is NOT a basis for staging.*

AJCC Cancer Staging Manual, Eighth Edition, Chapter 28 (Exocrine Pancreas) and Chapter 34 (Neuroendocrine Tumors of the Pancreas). This table has been amended for the context of this protocol and does not include all T Category options.

Note L: Intraoperative Lymph Node Findings, N Category

Explanatory Comments: In the context of intraoperative findings in this protocol for cancer surgery documentation, TNM categories from the American Joint Committee on Cancer (AJCC) are not designated with clinical (lower case "c" prefix) nor pathological (lower case "p" prefix) classifications. Determination of pathological classification involves a synthesis of information from multiple sources including clinical staging, operative findings, and pathological evaluation of resected surgical specimen(s). Complete information on TNM categories, clinical/pathological classifications, and the overall process of cancer staging can be found in the *AJCC Cancer Staging Manual, Eighth Edition.*

This field seeks to document intraoperative findings pertaining to nodal involvement and regional adenopathy. These findings help inform pathological classification (see Table 4). If regional adenopathy is suspected, response options are provided to indicate the completeness of resection. Information on lymphatic disease beyond normal regional drainage are considered metastatic and should be documented under **Intraoperative Metastatic Findings, M Category** (see Note M).

Table 4. Definition of Regional Lymph Node (N)

N Category	N Criteria (Exocrine Pancreas)	N Criteria (Neuroendocrine Tumors of the Pancreas)
NX	Regional lymph nodes cannot be assessed	Regional lymph nodes cannot be assessed
N0	No regional lymph node metastases	No regional lymph node involvement
N1	Metastasis in one to three regional lymph nodes	Regional lymph node involvement
N2	Metastasis in one to three regional lymph nodes	

AJCC Cancer Staging Manual, Eighth Edition, Chapter 28 (Exocrine Pancreas) and Chapter 34 (Neuroendocrine Tumors of the Pancreas).

Note M: Intraoperative Metastatic Findings, M Category

Explanatory Comments: In the context of intraoperative findings in this protocol for cancer surgery documentation, TNM categories from the American Joint Committee on Cancer (AJCC) are not designated with clinical (lower case "c" prefix) nor pathological (lower case "p" prefix) classifications. Determination of pathological classification involves a synthesis of information from multiple sources including clinical staging, operative findings, and pathological evaluation of resected surgical specimen(s). Complete information on TNM categories, clinical/pathological classifications, and the overall process of cancer staging can be found in the *AJCC Cancer Staging Manual, Eighth Edition*.

This field seeks to document intraoperative metastatic findings, which include nonregional adenopathy, peritoneal carcinomatosis, and metastasis to other organs. These findings help inform pathological classification (see Table 5).

Table 5. Definition of Distant Metastasis (M)

M Category	M Criteria (Exocrine Pancreas)	M Criteria (Neuroendocrine Tumors of the Pancreas)
M0	No distant metastasis	No distant metastasis
M1	Distant metastasis	Distant metastasis
M1a		Metastasis confined to liver
M1b		Metastases in at least one extrahepatic site (e.g., lung, ovary, nonregional lymph node, peritoneum, bone)
M1c		Both hepatic and extrahepatic metastases

AJCC Cancer Staging Manual, Eighth Edition, Chapter 28 (Exocrine Pancreas) and Chapter 34 (Neuroendocrine Tumors of the Pancreas).

Note N: Extrapancreatic Disease

Explanatory Comments: Common intraabdominal sites of metastatic disease include liver, peritoneum, and extraregional lymph nodes. If identified, select those that apply and describe if "Other" using the provided narrative box.

Note O: Assessment and Management of Vascular Involvement by Tumor

Explanatory Comments: Safe resection of tumors of the pancreas requires assessment and, if necessary, management of vascular involvement. Portal venous, superior mesenteric, and celiac branches may be involved on intraoperative assessment. The degree of involvement generally dictates management techniques; these can include dissection for separable disease or resection with (or without) reconstruction for inseparable disease, defined as tumor involvement with the vasculature that cannot be fully separated.

Select the vessels that were assessed and record the level of involvement for each. If inseparable, the surgeon should document the management of vascular involvement. Reconstruction options are listed with additional optional narrative fields so that additional information, such as the type of conduit, can be recorded.

Note P: Aberrant Arterial Anatomy

Explanatory Comments: Aberrant artery anatomy can be identified on preoperative imaging or intraoperative assessment. These often include replaced or accessory hepatic arteries. If identified, aberrant findings should be described in the provided narrative box.

Note Q: Completeness of Pancreatic Resection

Explanatory Comments: Documentation of residual gross disease is an important component of the operative report, given that only the surgeon can reliably distinguish an R1 margin from an R2 margin. R0/R1 should be indicated for cases when no gross tumor was left behind, irrespective of microscopic confirmation. An R2 response should be selected if there was macroscopic residual tumor, and a narrative box is provided to record additional details. Definitions for R Designation from the AJCC are summarized below in Table 6. For additional details, please refer to the *Operative Standards for Cancer Surgery*, Volume 1, page 193.

Table 6. Definition of R Designation (Residual Tumor After Treatment)

R	R Definition
R0	No residual tumor
R1	Microscopic residual tumor
R2	Macroscopic residual tumor at the primary cancer site or regional nodal sites (This designation is not used to indicate metastatic disease identified but not resected at surgical exploration.)

AJCC Cancer Staging Manual, Eighth Edition, Chapter 1 (Principles of Cancer Staging).

Note R: Intraoperative Margin Assessment

Explanatory Comments: Intraoperative evaluation of margin status should be performed and reported using a standard nomenclature following pancreatectomy. Options are provided to report the pancreatic parenchymal margin, bile duct margin, and uncinate (retroperitoneal/superior mesenteric artery) margin. Each margin that is assessed should be selected and either a positive or negative result should be reported. A "positive" response indicates that invasive cancer was found at the margin, whereas a "negative" response can be given for atypia or high-grade dysplasia. Additional margins can be reported using the "Other" response. The margin and result should be described in the associated narrative box.

For pancreatoduodenectomy, the pancreatic parenchymal margin, bile duct margin, and uncinate (retroperitoneal/superior mesenteric artery) margin should be reported by the surgeon. For distal subtotal pancreatectomy specimens, the pancreatic parenchymal margin should be reported. For total pancreatectomy specimens, the bile duct margin and uncinate (retroperitoneal/superior mesenteric artery) margin should be reported. For local excision/enucleation specimens, the pancreatic parenchymal margin may be reported. For additional details, please refer to the *Operative Standards for Cancer Surgery*, Volume 1, pages 191–196.

Note S: Additional Intraoperative Pathology Specimens

Explanatory Comments: Intraoperative staging can include excisional biopsy of indeterminate or suspicious lesions. Any additional pathology specimens assessed intraoperatively can be reported using this data item.

Note T: Procedure Performed

Explanatory Comments: Extent of surgical treatment needs to be clearly described. Options are provided for pancreatoduodenectomy (Whipple procedure), distal subtotal pancreatectomy, total pancreatectomy, or local excision/enucleation.

Pancreatoduodenectomy includes resection with or without partial gastrectomy ("classic" Whipple procedure or "pylorus preserving" Whipple procedure). Distal subtotal pancreatectomy includes resection with or without splenectomy. Total pancreatectomy includes resection of the pancreas and duodenum with or without partial gastrectomy. Local excision/enucleation is often the preferred surgical management for insulinoma and may be considered in select patients with low-risk pancreatic neuroendocrine tumors.

NCDB coding instructions for *Rx Summ—Surg 2023* [1291] are detailed in the STORE 2023 manual. Site-specific surgery codes for pancreas can be found in Appendix A and those relevant to this synoptic operative report are summarized below in Table 7.

Table 7. Relevant NCDB Site-Specific Surgery Codes for Pancreas Adapted from STORE Manual

NCDB Code	Definition
A250	Local excision of tumor, NOS
A300	Partial pancreatectomy, NOS; example: distal
A350	Local or partial pancreatectomy and duodenectomy
A360	WITHOUT distal/partial gastrectomy
A370	WITH partial gastrectomy (Whipple)
A400	Total pancreatectomy
A600	Total pancreatectomy and subtotal gastrectomy or duodenectomy

ACS Standards for Oncology Registry Entry (STORE) 2023. Appendix A: Site-Specific Surgery Codes, Pancreas.
* This table does not include codes A700 or A800 which fall outside the scope of this protocol.

Note U: Extent of Dissection and Lymphadenectomy

Explanatory Comments: If pancreatoduodenectomy was performed, the plane of uncinate (retroperitoneal/superior mesenteric artery) dissection, site of pancreatic transection, and extent of lymphadenectomy should be documented. For distal subtotal pancreatectomy, the plane of posterior dissection, site of pancreatic transection, and extent of lymphadenectomy should be documented. Total pancreatectomy procedures should document each of these except site of pancreatic transection. Local excision/enucleation should document preservation of the main pancreatic duct; if the main pancreatic duct is not preserved, additional surgical details should be documented using the provided narrative box. For any procedure, other noteworthy findings can be recorded using the provided narrative box.

Primary tumors of the proximal pancreas may infiltrate through the peripancreatic soft tissues into the perineural and lymphatic plexus surrounding vessels. Therefore, during pancreatoduodenectomy, the uncinate process should be dissected from the superior mesenteric artery along the periadventitial plane of the vessel, and the right lateral aspect of the vessel should be skeletonized from the level of the first jejunal branch of the superior mesenteric vein to the takeoff of the superior mesenteric artery from the aorta (see Figure 1). If dissection of the superior mesenteric artery margin along the periadventitial plane is not possible, a response of "alternate plane of retroperitoneal dissection" may be recorded. For additional details, please refer to the *Operative Standards for Cancer Surgery*, Volume 1, pages 207–211.

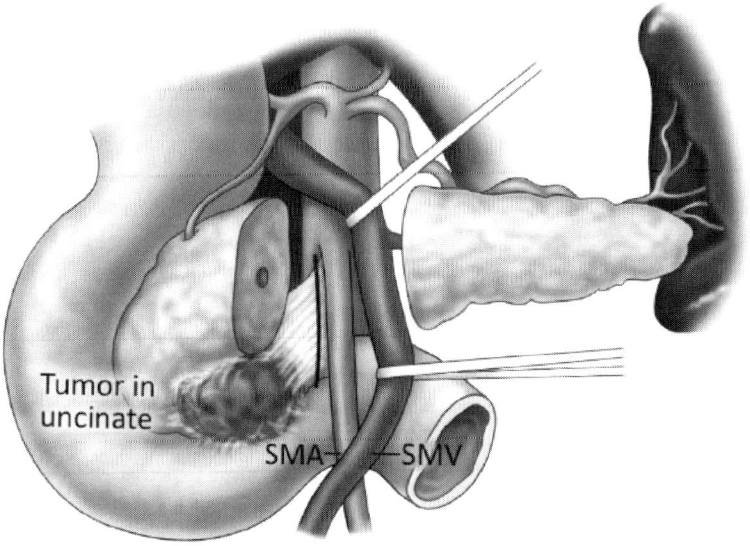

Figure 1. Resection of the uncinate process highlighting dissection along the periadventitial plane of the superior mesenteric artery.

In either a standard distal subtotal pancreatectomy or total pancreatectomy, posterior dissection is performed between the pancreas and anterior renal fascia with parenchymal transection just proximal to the site of disease (see Figure 2). A rim of grossly uninvolved soft tissue should be included both proximally and posteriorly. Alternate planes of posterior dissection, such as for the radical antegrade modular pancreatosplenectomy (RAMPS) procedure, can be documented as well. For additional details, please refer to the *Operative Standards for Cancer Surgery*, Volume 1, pages 242–244.

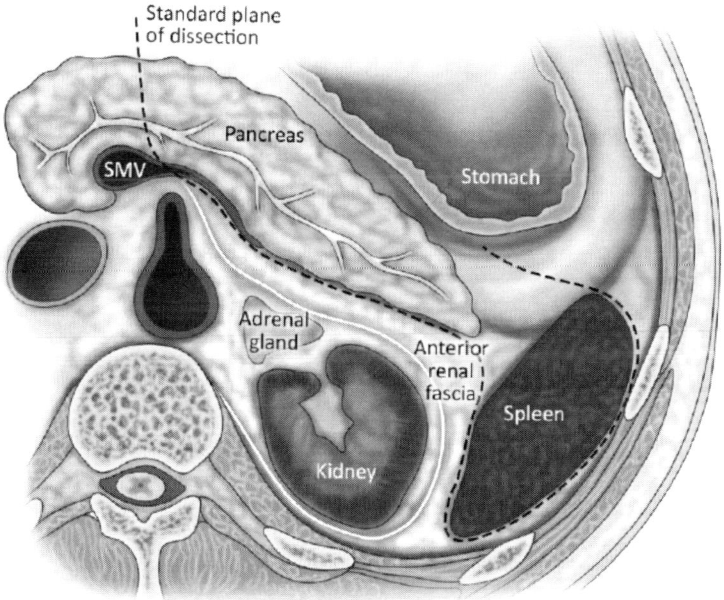

Figure 2. Resection of the pancreatic body and tail highlighting the standard plane of dissection along the anterior renal fascia. It may be necessary to resect adjacent retroperitoneal organs to remove all gross disease.

Whether for pancreatoduodenectomy or distal subtotal pancreatectomy, the pancreatic parenchyma should be transected so as to remove all gross disease within a normal-appearing gland. Depending on the tumor location, a more or less radical resection may be called for with transection at an alternate site of the pancreas. If transection was performed at a site other than the pancreatic neck, this should be described using the provided narrative box. For additional details, please refer to the *Operative Standards for Cancer Surgery*, Volume 1, pages 242–244.

Lymphadenectomy at the time of pancreatectomy is vital for obtaining staging information and to optimize local control. Standard lymphadenectomy for pancreatoduodenectomy includes the peripancreatic lymph nodes (head and uncinate; stations 13 and 17), the porta hepatis lymph nodes (stations 8 and 12), and the right lateral aspect of the superior mesenteric artery lymph nodes (station 14), as shown in Figure 3A. Standard lymphadenectomy for distal subtotal pancreatectomy includes the peripancreatic lymph nodes (body and tail; stations 11 and 18) and splenic hilum lymph nodes (station 10), as shown in Figure 3B. All aforementioned lymph node basins are included in the standard lymphadenectomy for total pancreatectomy, as shown in Figure 3C. Alternate lymphadenectomy (such as for local excision/enucleation procedures) should be documented by recording each nodal basin that was removed as part of the resection. For additional details, please refer to the *Operative Standards for Cancer Surgery*, Volume 1, pages 211–215 and 245–246.

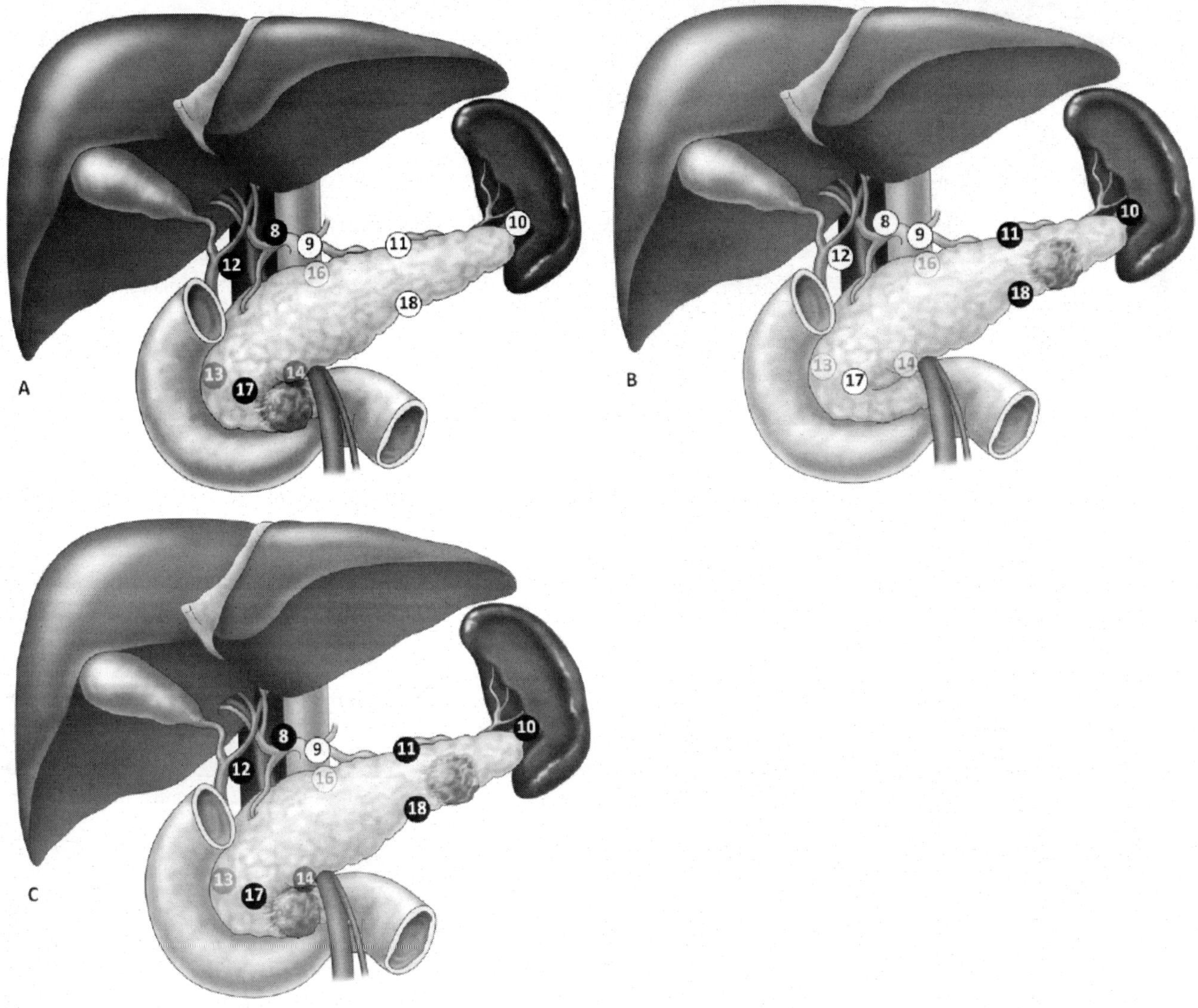

Figure 3. Standard lymphadenectomy for **(A)** pancreatoduodenectomy, **(B)** distal subtotal pancreatectomy, and **(C)** total pancreatectomy, with lymph node basins that should be resected shown in black for each procedure.

Section 3: Additional Procedure Details

Note V: Additional Procedure Details

Explanatory Comments: The following fields have been included for the synoptic operative report to represent a complete record of information so that it not only will fulfill surgeon and institutional documentation needs, but also can fulfill regulatory requirements. The inclusion of open-text narrative fields provides sufficient flexibility for all aspects of surgical care to be recorded and for multiple functions, such as registry submission and generation of billing codes, to be permissible.

Note W: Staging Laparoscopy Performed

Explanatory Comments: Staging laparoscopy should be considered to assess for intraabdominal metastasis, especially when it is likely to alter the surgical plan. This decision is at the discretion of the surgeon but may be influenced by several factors including clinical tumor stage, laboratory testing, or preoperative imaging. For additional details, please refer to the *Operative Standards for Cancer Surgery*, Volume 1, pages 187–191.

Note X: Operative Approach

Explanatory Comments: Several technical approaches to pancreatectomy are now available for the surgical removal of the primary tumor and regional lymph nodes, including minimally invasive and open laparotomy procedures. Selection of the approach may be based on the patient and surgeon preference or other clinical factors. Use the narrative box to explain any circumstances outside of the options provided. Relevant NCDB codes are provided in Table 8 for the *Approach – Surgery of the Primary Site at this Facility (RxHospSurgApp 2010)* [668] data item from STORE 2023.

Table 8. Relevant NCDB Codes for *Approach – Surgery of the Primary Site at this Facility* from STORE Manual

NCDB Code	Label
0	No surgical procedure of primary site at this facility; Diagnosed at autopsy
1	Robotic assisted
2	Robotic converted to open
3	Minimally invasive (such as endoscopic or laparoscopic)
4	Minimally invasive (endoscopic or laparoscopic) converted to open
5	Open or approach unspecified

ACS Standards for Oncology Registry Entry (STORE) 2023. Approach – Surgery of the Primary Site at this Facility (RxHospSurgApp 2010).
*This table has been amended to remove code 9 (Unknown whether the surgery was performed at this facility) as it would not be an appropriate code in the context of this report.

Note Y: Cholecystectomy

Explanatory Comments: Cholecystectomy is often performed at the time of pancreatic or biliary tract surgery. Please indicate whether cholecystectomy was performed.

Note Z: Extent of Gastric Resection

Explanatory Comments: Cancer operations that remove the head of the pancreas also include removal of the duodenum. Depending on the location and extent of the tumor, as well as surgeon and patient preferences, the antrum of the stomach may be included in the resection, or the pylorus and stomach may be preserved. Documentation should include whether classic resection (with distal gastrectomy) or pylorus preserving resection was performed.

Note AA: Orientation of Reconstruction

Explanatory Comments: Following surgical removal of the pancreatic head, the surgeon has a range of options for reconstruction of the gastrointestinal tract, biliary tree, and remnant pancreas (when needed). Please indicate whether loop (Billroth II type), Roux-en-Y, or other orientation of reconstruction was performed, and enter additional details in the associated narrative box.

Note BB: Pancreatic Reconstruction

Explanatory Comments: Following pancreatic resection, the surgeon has a range of options for pancreatic reconstruction. Please indicate whether pancreaticojejunostomy, pancreaticogastrostomy, or other form of pancreatic reconstruction was performed. In addition, please provide a description of the surgical technique. Additional technical details about the procedure can be entered in the narrative box, as needed.

Note CC: Biliary Reconstruction

Explanatory Comments: Following surgical removal of the pancreatic head, surgeons commonly perform a one-layer duct-to-mucosa anastomosis for biliary reconstruction, although other techniques may be performed based on surgeon preference. Please provide additional technical details about the procedure in the narrative box, as needed.

Note DD: Intestinal Reconstruction

Explanatory Comments: Following pancreatectomy, reconstruction of the gastrointestinal tract is often required, for which the surgeon has a range of options. Please select whether gastrojejunostomy, duodenojejunostomy, or other reconstruction was performed. Additional technical details about the procedure can be entered in the narrative box, as needed.

Note EE: Splenectomy

Explanatory Comments: Splenectomy is often performed at the time of pancreatic surgery. Please indicate whether splenectomy was performed.

Note FF: Method of Pancreatic Transection

Explanatory Comments: The surgeon has a range of options by which to transect the pancreas during pancreatectomy. This can be performed through use of a stapler or with other surgical devices. Please select whether a non-stapled, stapled, or other approach was used and provide additional technical details about the procedure in the narrative box, as needed.

Note GG: Management of Pancreatic 'Stump'

Explanatory Comments: Following pancreatic resection, there are a range of options by which to manage the transected pancreas. Surgeons commonly use sutures or staples on the pancreatic stump. Please select whether one of these approaches was performed and provide additional technical details about the procedure in the narrative box, as needed.

Note HH: Drains

Explanatory Comments: Post-operative pancreatic fistula is a common complication of pancreatic surgery. Surgical drains can be used to detect or manage pancreatic fistula or other causes of intraabdominal infection. Please indicate whether a surgical drain was used and enter additional detail about drain type, location, etc. in the narrative box, as needed.

Note II: Stents

Explanatory Comments: Surgeons may use stents to reduce the likelihood of anastomotic leak or to improve rates of anastomotic patency following pancreatic surgery. Please indicate whether a stent was used and enter additional detail about stent type, location, etc., in the narrative box, as needed.

Note JJ: Additional Procedures

Explanatory Comments: Whether to perform additional surgeries should be individualized based on risk and benefits, and those details can be documented here. Similarly, adjacent organs may be removed, or additional procedures may be performed at the surgeon's discretion in the management of the patient's cancer. Details can be recorded in the narrative box, as needed.

Note KK: Additional Surgical Information

Explanatory Comments: While concordance with operative standards has been the primary focus of this synoptic operative report, end user focus groups requested the scope of the tool to be expanded in order for it to comply with all surgical reporting requirements. As a result, this report can now be considered a comprehensive operative report and it can be used to help generate billing codes and output data into hospital registries.

There was not sufficient consensus, however, on non-cancer surgical information, such as patient positioning, incision location, port placement, fascial closure, etc., and so narrative text options are provided for inserting information the surgeon considers important.

Note LL: Intraoperative Complications

Explanatory Comments: Intraoperative complications are rare, but important to document them regardless of whether they are related to focal surgical difficulties or systemic events that may relate to patient positioning, delivery of anesthesia, or other aspects of the surgical procedure.

References

1. Amin MB, Edge SB, Greene FL, et al, eds. *AJCC Cancer Staging Manual*. 8th ed. New York, NY: Springer; 2017.
2. National Comprehensive Cancer Network. NCCN Guidelines for Pancreatic Adenocarcinoma (Version 1.2022). https://www.nccn.org/professionals/physician_gls/pdf/pancreatic.pdf. Accessed April 26, 2022.
3. Commission on Cancer. *Standards for Oncology Registry Entry (STORE)*. Chicago, IL: American College of Surgeons; 2023.
4. Nelson H, Hunt KK, Veeramachaneni N, et al. *Operative Standards for Cancer Surgery*. Vol 1. Chicago, IL: Wolters Kluwer; 2015.

Made in United States
North Haven, CT
05 November 2026

21767742R00017